Medical Emergencies in Early Childhood Settings

Emergency Telephone Numbers

Emergency Medical Services (EMS): _____

Poison Center: _800-222-1222_____

Police Department: _____

Fire Department: _____

Health Consultant: _____

Physician: _____

Dentist: _____

Hospital: _____

Other: _____

When in doubt of whom to call, dial 911.

In most communities, dialing 911 will access local emergency services. However, some communities do not have 911 access, and some cellular phone services do not automatically access the closest emergency services. The direct phone numbers for your local emergency services should be posted by the phone.

All early care and education (ECE) staff members should be familiar with the Emergency Medical Services (EMS) in their community *before* they are actually needed for an emergency. Find out the answers to the following questions:

- What is the best telephone number to reach EMS?
- How fast will emergency help arrive?
- What hospital do they use? How long will it take to transport a child to the hospital?
- What authorization or documentation is required for them to treat and/or transport a child?
- May a staff member accompany the child to the hospital?

Familiarize children with emergency personnel and other community helpers as part of your early childhood curriculum. For curriculum suggestions and children's learning activities, check out *Growing, Growing Strong: A Whole Health Curriculum for Young Children* (Redleaf Press, 2006).

Contents

Contents

Foreword

Dr. Donald Palmer

This book is written for you, the caregiver. Its purpose is to provide you with a quick and accurate reference for appropriate action during medical emergencies occurring in the early care and education (ECE) setting. Take some time to familiarize yourself with the information in and organization of this book so you can use it effectively if needed during an emergency situation.

First aid is the immediate care given to a person who has been injured or suddenly becomes ill, in order to stabilize and possibly address the situation until medical help is obtained as indicated. First aid in the ECE setting may involve something as simple as washing and bandaging a scratched knee, or it may mean performing abdominal thrusts to clear a blocked airway.

All staff members who are involved in providing direct care for children should have training in pediatric first aid, including management of a blocked airway and administration of rescue breathing.

The provision of first aid should be thoughtful, orderly, and rapid. During an emergency, first evaluate the situation. Find out what happened and who is involved. Quickly inspect the child who is injured or ill with a "hands off" approach (without touching the child). Evaluate the child's ABCs: **A**ppearance, **B**reathing, and **C**irculation. You should complete the ABCs in 30 seconds or less.

After this brief appraisal, be sure noninvolved children are adequately supervised and out of the way.

Quickly return to the child to perform a "hands on" evaluation. Does Emergency Medical Services (EMS) need to be called? What first aid actions can you give?

After these steps are completed, notify the child's parent or guardian. Comfort the ill or injured child, explain what has happened, and answer questions. Write a thorough incident report.

Remember that prevention is the first, best form of treatment.

Dr. Palmer is nationally recognized for his expertise and efforts to promote child health. Some of his accomplishments include being a member of the American Academy of Pediatrics (AAP) Committee on Early Childhood, Adoption, and Dependent Care; a reviewer of Caring for Our Children; *a member of the Steering Committee for Pediatric First Aid for Caregivers and Teachers; a certified playground inspector; a member of the AAP Committee on Injury, Violence, and Poison Prevention; and the former president of the Alabama Chapter of AAP.*

Standard Precautions

Most medical emergency situations in ECE settings are not life-threatening. These situations allow you time to wash your hands, put on gloves, and access first aid supplies. By following simple practices known as "standard precautions," you can help reduce the spread of infection and prevent transmission of blood-borne germs such as those that cause HIV/AIDS or hepatitis B.

Follow standard precautions in all medical emergencies or situations involving first aid or medical care. These procedures will help protect you, the injured or ill child, and other children and adults in the environment. The basics of standard precautions are:

- Wash hands with soap and running water.
- Wear non-porous, disposable, non-latex gloves.
- Carefully clean up spills that may contain blood or other body fluids.
- Clean contaminated surfaces.
- Sanitize (disinfect) contaminated surfaces.
- Properly discard used gloves, bandages, tissues, and so on.
- Wash hands again after removing gloves.

Hand Washing

- Wash hands with liquid soap and running water. Lather well, then rub hands for **at least** 10 seconds. Clean the wrists, palms, fingers, in between fingers, back of hands, and around fingernails.
- Liquid hand sanitizers (waterless soaps) and premoistened wipes **are not** an effective substitute for soap and running water. However, if soap and running water are not available (when transporting children or during nature walks, for example) the first aid responder should remove dirt from her hands with the wipes, and then apply liquid sanitizer using the following procedure.
  » Apply a generous amount of hand sanitizer into the palm of one hand.
  » Rub hands together until sanitizer covers fingers, palms, and wrists. Hands should be completely covered.
  » Let sanitizer air-dry.

Non-Latex Gloves

- Because of possible allergic reaction, always use non-latex gloves.
- Maintain an ample supply of single-use, non-porous, disposable non-latex gloves. Gloves should be powder-free.
- Gloves must be available **at all times** when children are present.
- Gloves must be discarded after one use. **Never** use gloves twice.
- Hands must be washed **before** putting on gloves, and **after** gloves are removed.

Cleaning and Sanitizing

Cleaning removes visible spills, dirt, debris, and so on. Clean all surfaces, including outdoor surfaces, possibly contaminated with blood or other body fluids (including vomit, urine, stool, and saliva).

- Wear non-porous gloves.
- Clean up the spill using paper towels, tissues, or rags. Use disposables if possible.
- Put soiled towels or rags into a plastic-lined receptacle for disposal or to launder/ sanitize later.
- Use soapy water to clean all surfaces.
- Rinse the surface with water.
- Sanitize surface.

Sanitizing (disinfecting) kills germs including bacteria, viruses, and fungi. A mild bleach solution is one of the most effective disinfectants.

- Mix fresh bleach solution each day. Old solution cannot kill germs. The solution "recipe" is based on using regular bleach, not "ultra" bleach.
- Bleach disinfecting solution for use in bathrooms and diapering areas:
  » 1 tablespoon bleach + 1 quart water, **or**
  » ¼ cup bleach + 1 gallon water
- Bleach disinfecting solution for use on toys, eating utensils, table surfaces, and so on:
  » 1 tablespoon bleach + 1 gallon water
- Store bleach solution in a clearly labeled spray bottle.
- Keep bleach and bleach solution out of children's reach.

TO SANITIZE SURFACES:

- Wear non-porous gloves.
- Apply sanitizing solution to surfaces **after** cleaning up visible dirt and spills.
- Wet surface thoroughly with the solution and let air-dry.
- If surface must be wiped dry, allow solution to remain on surface for 2 minutes before wiping dry.
- Properly dispose of towel or cloth used to wipe surface.
- Store sanitizing solution out of children's reach.
- Remove gloves, and then wash hands.

Planning and Preparation

Staff Training

All staff members should have training in dealing with medical emergencies. Along with general training in basic first aid, more specific training is also recommended.

- At least one staff person who is currently certified in pediatric first aid (including CPR) must be available on site at all times and in all places where children are present.
- All staff members, substitute staff members, and volunteers involved in providing direct care for children should have up-to-date training in the following areas:
  » Pediatric first aid, including management of a blocked airway (choking) and rescue breathing
  » Sanitation and standard precautions
  » Child safety and injury prevention

- At least one staff member who is currently certified in pediatric CPR must be immediately available when children are involved in swimming and wading.
- At least one staff member who is currently certified in pediatric CPR must be immediately available when a child is known to have a specific special health need (such as cardiac arrhythmia) that makes the child more likely than a typical child to require cardiac resuscitation.
- Staff members directly responsible for children with special health care needs should be trained in administration of all medical procedures and/or medications that might be required for that child (an epinephrine auto-injector, for example). Training should be provided by a qualified health care professional.
- Program directors should regularly review caregivers' ability to perform first aid and to respond to medical emergencies.
- Fully stocked first aid kits and children's life-sustaining medicines (such as epinephrine auto-injectors) must be clearly marked and immediately available to the caregiver at all times, including on trips outside the facility.
- Caregivers should have immediate access to communication (such as cellular phones) at all times and in all places where children are in care.

Authorization and Documentation

Maintain current documentation on each child. Update the following information regularly according to your licensing regulations:

- Names of parents, guardians, or other people who can authorize medical treatment
- Signed authorization forms, including all forms required under HIPAA (Health Insurance Portability and Accountability Act), such as Release of Information forms
- Names of family members and other emergency contacts and current phone numbers
- Names and phone numbers of each child's physician, dentist, and preferred hospital
- List of any allergies
- Diagnosis and treatment, including emergency care plan, for children with special health care needs, including specific indications for use and dose for any medications

Document all instances of illness or injury, no matter how minor, and the treatment provided. Provide specific details for every event.

First Aid Kit

A first aid kit should be readily available wherever children are in care, including during field trips, when playing outdoors, and while being transported.

- First aid supplies must be stored in a clearly marked, closed container.
- A first aid kit must be accessible to child caregivers, but out of children's reach.
- Restock the kit after each use.
- Include a checklist of items inside the kit. Check and document inventory monthly; replace missing or unusable items.
- **Do not** include any medications in the kit unless prescribed for a specific child (such as an epinephrine auto-injector).
- Do not store the kit in a hot vehicle or leave in direct heat.

RECOMMENDED ITEMS:

- Disposable, non-porous, non-latex gloves
- Liquid soap
- Premoistened cloths and hand sanitizer (if water is not available to wash hands)
- Tweezers
- Ear thermometer or other non-glass digital thermometer (with instructions)
- Adhesive strip bandages (assorted sizes)
- Sterile gauze pads
- Flexible roller gauze
- Bandage tape
- Safety pins
- Eye shield
- Triangular bandages
- Small plastic or metal splints
- Any prescribed emergency medication needed for a specific child (such as an epinephrine auto-injector)
- Sterile water
- Plastic zipper bags (assorted sizes)
- Bandage scissors
- Current standard first aid chart, first aid guide, and a copy of this Redleaf Quick Guide
- Pen/pencil and note pad
- Cellular phone, or coins or phone card for use in a pay phone
- Telephone numbers of Poison Center, paramedics, and other emergency services
- List of home, cellular, and work phone numbers for parents, family members, or emergency contact person for each child
- Plastic bags to dispose of contaminated supplies

ADDITIONAL ITEMS AND RECOMMENDATIONS for first aid supplies:

- Cold packs
  - » "Instant" cold packs are useful in first aid kits, especially kits available during transportation, on field trips, or while playing outdoors.
  - » Cold packs can be made by putting ice in a plastic bag or wrapping ice in a cloth.
  - » A closed bag of frozen vegetables can be used as a cold pack.
  - » **Do not** place ice or a cold pack directly on a child's skin. A cold pack or ice can injure skin and tissue (frostnip) if placed directly on the skin. Always wrap ice or cold pack in a cloth, or place a cloth or thick gauze over the child's skin before applying the ice or cold pack.
- The Save-A-Tooth and EMT ToothSaver systems include appropriate supplies in case a tooth is knocked out.
- Disposable mouth guards or CPR barriers may be included for rescue breathing.
- A bottle of sterile, non-preserved ophthalmic saline solution can be included in the first aid kit and used to flush eyes. Solution is for one-time use only. Any unused solution must be disposed of and replaced with an unopened bottle.
- Activated charcoal is sometimes used after a poison has been ingested. It should be administered only with instruction from the Poison Center or a physician and ideally with parental knowledge and permission.

AN ABBREVIATED FIRST AID KIT containing essential items may be more practical for playground or outside activities taking place near the facility. Supplies may be carried in a clearly marked fanny pack worn by a staff member.

- Disposable, non-porous, non-latex gloves
- Premoistened cloths and hand sanitizer (if water is not available to wash hands)
- Tweezers
- Adhesive strip bandages (assorted sizes)
- Sterile gauze pads
- Flexible roller gauze
- Bandage tape
- Any prescribed emergency medication needed for specific children (such as an epinephrine auto-injector)
- Instant cold pack
- Cloth to protect skin from cold pack
- Plastic zipper bags (assorted sizes)
- Scissors
- Pen/pencil and note pad
- Telephone numbers of Poison Center, paramedics, and other emergency services
- Plastic bags to dispose of contaminated supplies

Bleeding

If a child or adult is injured and is bleeding, control of bleeding is a priority. Life-threatening amounts of blood can be lost very quickly.

- Determine where the blood is coming from, and whether bleeding has stopped.
  - » Call EMS if any steady or "pulsing" bleeding is not easily controlled within a few minutes.
  - » Some superficial wounds, such as those on the scalp, tend to bleed profusely but generally are not life-threatening.

Controlling Bleeding

- Put on non-latex gloves.
- If possible, lay the child down and give comfort/reassurance.
- Remove any loose debris from the wound. **Do not** attempt to remove an object imbedded in a deep wound, including glass. This may lead to more bleeding. Instead, place bandages around the object to secure object in place.
- Place gauze or other clean material on the wound.
- Apply direct pressure with your fingers or palm of your hand to the area that is bleeding. Continue pressure until the bleeding stops (usually 1 to 2 minutes). *See figure 1.*
- If blood soaks through, place additional gauze on top of the first compress. **Do not** remove the original compress.
- If possible, and no other injury (such as a fracture or head injury) is suspected, elevate the injured part of the body so it is above the level of the child's heart.

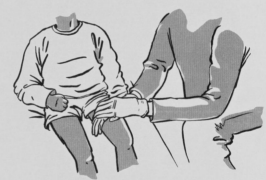

figure 1

CALL EMS IF:

- Bleeding is severe or appears to be arterial (bright red, spurting or pulsing flow).
- Bleeding does not stop with 5 minutes of continuous direct pressure. Continue to apply pressure until EMS personnel arrive. **Do not** apply a tourniquet.
- The child is bleeding from the head.
- A body part is crushed, or partially or fully amputated.
  - » Keep the amputated body part clean.
  - » Wrap the body part with wet gauze using sterile water and place in a plastic bag.
  - » Keep the body part *with the child.*
- An object is embedded deep within the wound.
- The child shows symptoms of **shock**. *See the section on Shock under "SUDDEN ILLNESS" for more information.*

- Internal injury or bleeding is suspected. Symptoms can include the following:
  - » The child complains of severe pain.
  - » The child appears very ill (pale, weak, clammy, fainting).
  - » Soft tissues (such as in the abdomen) are tender, swollen, or hard.
  - » The child has a rapid, weak pulse.
  - » The child has nausea or vomiting, or is vomiting blood.
  - » The child has bruising extending from the injured area.

Contact the child's family.

Nosebleed

- Put on non-latex gloves.
- Help the child sit up with head tilted slightly forward. *See figure 2.*
- Pinch the nostrils closed. Apply gentle pressure for at least 5 minutes.
- If possible, apply a cloth-wrapped cold pack to the child's nose and cheeks while applying pressure.
- Gently release the nose. If bleeding starts again, reapply the pressure for 10 minutes.
- After the nosebleed stops, gently clean any blood from the child's face and skin; provide clean clothing if necessary.
- Discourage the child from blowing or picking his nose. Have the child do a quiet activity for at least 30 minutes.

CALL EMS IF:

- The nosebleed cannot easily be controlled after 15 minutes.
- It is accompanied by dizziness or weakness.
- It occurs after a blow to the head or a fall.

Contact the child's family if EMS has been called.

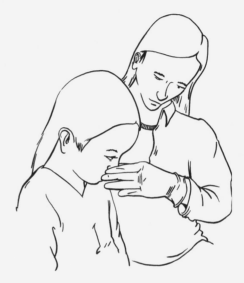

figure 2

Wounds, Cuts, and Blisters

Open Wounds

- Put on non-latex gloves.
- Control the bleeding with direct pressure. *See "BLEEDING" for more information.*
- Contact the child's family and recommend **immediate medical attention** if the wound:
  - » Does not stop bleeding after 5 minutes or more of direct pressure.
  - » Appears deep.
  - » Will not stay closed by itself or if a cut or wound is longer than 1/2 inch.
  - » Is on the face, or involves the eyes or ears.
  - » Is on the lip and crosses onto the cheek.
  - » Is from a bite (animal or human). *See "BITES AND STINGS" for more information.*
- For minor wounds (cuts, scratches, and scrapes), once the bleeding stops, gently wash the wound with soap and water, then apply a clean dressing and bandage.

Puncture Wounds

Puncture wounds may be either deep (such as a knife wound) or shallow (such as a splinter or nail). These wounds generally do not bleed much; however, deep puncture wounds can be serious.

- Put on non-latex gloves.
- If the object is small and can be easily removed (such as a nail or thumbtack that has been stepped on), then remove the object.
- Allow the wound to bleed freely for a few minutes to help remove debris.
- After a few minutes, control bleeding with direct pressure. *See "BLEEDING" for more information.*
- Once bleeding stops, gently wash the wound with soap and water.
- Apply a clean dressing and bandage.
- Contact the child's family and recommend they consult their doctor's office for further instruction and to confirm tetanus booster status.

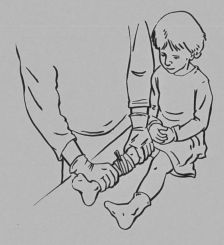

figure 3

CALL EMS IF:

- The penetrating object is large or deeply embedded (such as glass, a stick, or a knife).
  - » **Do not** remove objects that are protruding (sticking out). Removal could cause further internal damage and severe bleeding.
  - » Hold the child still in order to immobilize the object. Place bandages around the object to secure object in place or hold the object still until EMS personnel arrive. *See figure 3.*

Contact child's family if EMS has been called.

Splinters/Slivers

If the splinter is small and is sticking out of the skin, it probably can be easily removed.

- Clean tweezers with soap and water.
- Put on non-latex gloves.
- Grasp the splinter with tweezers. Gently pull the splinter out from the opposite direction that it went into the skin.
- **Do not** use a needle or other invasive procedure to remove splinters.
- After the splinter is removed, gently wash the wound with soap and water.
- Apply a clean dressing and bandage, if needed.
- Inform the child's family that you removed a splinter.

If the splinter is large or deeply embedded, or if you cannot easily remove the entire splinter with clean tweezers, then seek medical attention.

Blisters

- Put on non-latex gloves.
- Protect blisters with a clean bandage. **Do not** break blisters.
- Contact the child's family and recommend medical attention if the blister is larger than the size of a quarter or if there are multiple blisters.

PRESCRIPTION FOR PREVENTION

- Check outdoor play areas each day and remove trash, sticks, glass, or other debris.
- Regularly inspect wooden play equipment for splinters; repair as needed.

Rescue Breathing

Call EMS if a child shows any problems
with breathing.

A child who is not breathing can sustain
brain damage or die very quickly.

Opening the Airway

- If a head or neck injury is **not** suspected, use the
  head-tilt/chin-lift method. *See figure 4.*
  - » Place your hand on the child's forehead. Tilt head back
    slightly.
  - » Place fingers of your other hand under the child's chin. Lift
    gently.
  - » **Do not** use your thumb to lift the jaw; use your fingers.
  - » **Do not** press on the neck or soft tissue under the jaw.

- If a head or neck injury **is** suspected, use the *jaw-lift* method.
  See figure 5.
  - » Stabilize the head. **Do not** move or tilt head.
  - » Place your fingers behind the angles of the child's lower jaw on each side.
  - » Gently push the lower jaw forward.

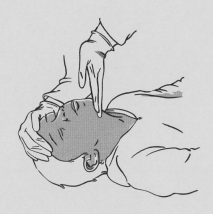

figure 4

Performing Rescue Breathing

Rescue breathing involves forcing air into the child's body.

- Check for responsiveness. Tap the infant's foot, or rub the child,
  and shout "Are you okay?"
- Open the airway using the head-tilt/chin-lift or the jaw-lift
  method.
- Look, listen, and feel for breathing. Position yourself so your ear is
  over the child's mouth and nose:
  - » Look to see if the chest and abdomen are rising and falling
    with breaths.
  - » Listen for breath.

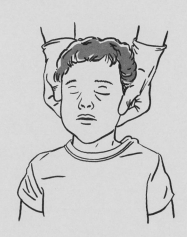

figure 5

- » Feel for breath on your ear and cheek.
- » Take 5 to 10 seconds to do this.
- Put on non-latex gloves.
- If there is no breathing, look in the mouth for any object blocking breathing.
  - » If the object is easy to remove with fingers, carefully remove it.
  - » Do not attempt to remove an object deep in the throat.
  - » Do not attempt a blind "finger sweep" of the mouth.
- If there is no breathing, begin rescue breathing.
- Use a CPR breathing barrier (for example, a face shield or resuscitation mask) or mouth guard over the child's mouth and/or nose.

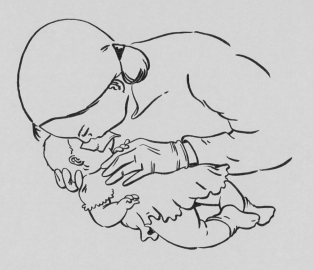

figure 6

  - » **Infant**: Cover the infant's mouth and nose with the breathing barrier. Breathe gently into the valve of the breathing barrier. *See figure 6.*
  - » **Toddler or older child**: Cover the child's mouth and nose with the breathing barrier. Breathe gently into the valve of the breathing barrier.
- Follow this procedure.
  - » Give 2 slow breaths, enough so you can see the chest rise and fall.
  - » If chest does not rise and fall, reposition the head and/or jaw to open the airway, and repeat breaths.
  - » Allow the air to flow out of the chest between breaths. Check for breathing.
- Look, listen, and feel for breathing. If there is no breathing, begin alternating chest compressions *(see section on Chest Compressions below for instructions)* and breaths.
  - » Give 5 chest compressions.
  - » Check the mouth for any object blocking breathing.
  - » Give 1 rescue breath.
  - » Repeat, alternating 30 chest compressions, checking mouth, and 2 breaths.
- Continue until the child begins breathing or EMS arrives.

Chest Compressions

Chest compression performed properly compresses the heart, pumping blood and oxygen throughout the body until the heart resumes beating.

INFANT—Chest Compression

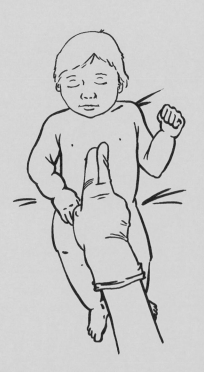

- Place the infant on his back on a firm, flat surface.
- Place 2 fingers (index and middle fingers) on the infant's breastbone at the nipple line, and above the bottom tip of the breastbone. *See figure 7.*
- Give 5 chest thrusts in rapid succession, pushing the breastbone down approximately 1/3 of the chest depth.

figure 7

- Check the mouth for any object blocking breathing.
- Give 1 rescue breath.
- Repeat, alternating 30 chest compressions with 2 breaths. Continue until the infant begins breathing or EMS arrives.

TODDLER AND OLDER CHILD—Chest Compression

- Place the child on his back on a firm, flat surface.
- Place the heel of your hand on the child's breastbone slightly below the nipple line, but above the bottom tip of the breastbone. *See figure 8.*
- Give 5 chest thrusts in rapid succession, pushing the breastbone down approximately 1 to 1-1/2 inches.
- Check the mouth for any object blocking breathing.
- Give 1 rescue breath.
- Repeat, alternating 30 chest compressions with 2 breaths. Continue until the child begins breathing or EMS arrives.

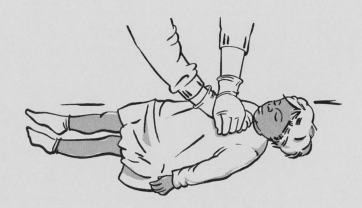

figure 8

Asthma or Chronic Respiratory Condition

If a child has been diagnosed with asthma or other chronic respiratory condition:

- ECE staff should work with the child's parents and health care professionals to develop an emergency care plan or asthma action plan.
- Any prescribed medications or supplies (such as peak flow meters, quick-acting inhalers, spacers, or epinephrine auto-injectors) must be kept near the child at all times. Medications must be properly stored and out of children's reach.
- Caregivers directly involved in the care of the child should have specific training related to the child's condition, including how to manage an acute asthma attack (or other respiratory-related emergency) and how to administer medications.
- Other staff members involved in the care of the child should be aware of the condition and that there is an emergency care plan.
- Some state laws allow licensed child care providers to administer inhaled medication for respiratory problems such as asthma. Check your local licensing regulations and follow procedures established by signed parental medical authorization.

IN CASE OF AN ASTHMA EPISODE OR OTHER RESPIRATORY DISTRESS:

- Follow the child's emergency care plan or asthma action plan.
- Use a quick-acting inhaled medication only if it has been prescribed for that child.
- Observe the child's breathing. If normal breathing does not resume within 10 minutes, follow the emergency care plan, including cailing EMS.
- If child is not breathing, begin rescue breathing.

Near-Drowning and Drowning

- Call EMS.
- Remove child from water.
- Remove any obvious blockage (such as seaweed or mud) from his mouth.
- Check breathing.
- If child is not breathing, begin rescue breathing.

Strangulation or Suffocation

- Call EMS.
- Remove object (cord, pillow, plastic, soft mattress).
- Check breathing.
- If child is not breathing, begin rescue breathing.

PRₓESCRIPTION FOR PREVENTION

The directions for CPR rescue breathing and chest compression are revised and updated often. It is wise to check the Web site of the American Heart Association (www.americanheart.org), the American Red Cross (www.redcross.org), or the Mayo Clinic (www.mayoclinic.com) regularly to make sure you are familiar with the latest methods.

Choking

- Observe child for symptoms of choking.
- Call EMS. If you are alone, provide 1 minute of lifesaving first aid care, and then call EMS.
- If the child is coughing:
  - » Encourage coughing. It is the best way to remove a blockage.
  - » **Do not** pat the child on the back.
  - » **Do not** hold up the child's arms or hold child upside down.
- Look inside the child's mouth.
- If object is easy to remove with your fingers, carefully remove it.
  - » **Do not** "finger sweep" the mouth to remove the object. You might push it in deeper.
- If the object is **not** removed and/or the child stops breathing, follow the procedures for "Infant Choking" and "Toddler or Older Child Choking" below.

Infant Choking (1 year of age and younger)

If infant is **responsive** (conscious) and not breathing:

- Administer a combination of 5 back blows and 5 chest thrusts.
- Back blows:
  - » Lay the infant face down on your forearm, with the infant's feet up toward your shoulder.
  - » Place your hand around the infant's jaw and neck for support.
  - » Rest your arm against your thigh for support. Use the heel of your other hand to give 5 quick, sharp back blows between the infant's shoulder blades.
  - » If object does not fall out of infant's mouth, give 5 chest thrusts.
- Chest thrusts: *See figure 9.*
  - » Turn infant chest up, resting on your forearm.
  - » Support arm against your thigh. The infant's head should be lower than your trunk.
  - » Place 2 fingers (index and middle fingers) from your other hand on the infant's breastbone slightly below the nipple line, but above the bottom tip of the breastbone.
  - » Give 5 chest thrusts in rapid succession, pushing the breastbone down approximately $\frac{1}{2}$ to 1 inch.

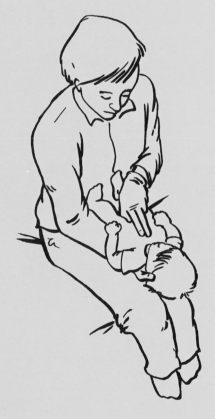

figure 9

- Put on non-latex gloves and check inside the infant's mouth after you do the chest thrusts. If you see the object causing the choking, carefully remove it. Then observe the infant's breathing. Perform rescue breathing if needed. *See "RESCUE BREATHING" for more information.*
- If the object is not removed, continue alternating back blows, chest thrusts, and checking mouth until EMS arrives, or the object is removed, or the child becomes unresponsive.

If infant is **not responsive** (becomes unconscious) and not breathing, follow rescue breathing procedure. *See "RESCUE BREATHING" for more information.*

- Check for responsiveness.
- Open the airway.
- Look, listen, and feel for breathing.
- Put on non-latex gloves, and look in mouth for an object. Remove it if possible.
- Begin rescue breathing.
- If the infant does not start to breathe after opening the airway:
  - » Begin 30 chest compressions.
  - » Check mouth.
  - » Give 2 rescue breaths.
  - » Repeat until the infant begins to breathe or EMS arrives.

Toddler or Older Child Choking

If child is **responsive** (conscious) and not breathing:

- Administer abdominal thrusts.
  - » Stand or kneel behind the child. Pull the child close to you.
  - » Make a fist and place it just above the child's navel, and below the breastbone.
  - » Cover your fist with your other hand, and give a quick upward and inward thrust to the child's abdomen.
- Continue abdominal thrusts until EMS arrives, the object is removed, or the child becomes unresponsive.

If the child is **not responsive** (becomes unconscious) and not breathing, follow rescue breathing procedures. *See "RESCUE BREATHING" for more information.*

- Check for responsiveness.
- Open the airway.
- Look, listen, and feel for breathing.
- Put on non-latex gloves, and look in mouth for an object. Remove it if possible.
- Begin rescue breathing.
- If the child does not start to breathe after opening the airway:
  - » Begin 30 chest compressions.
  - » Check mouth.
  - » Give 2 rescue breaths.
  - » Repeat until the child begins to breathe or EMS arrives.

PRₓESCRIPTION FOR PREVENTION

- Avoid serving foods that are potential choking hazards, such as hot dogs, popcorn, and hard candy.
- Empty all containers, such as wading pools or buckets, when not in use. Never leave standing water unattended.
- **Do not** allow latex balloons or plastic dry cleaning bags in the ECE environment.

Poisoning

Poisons can affect the body quickly!

CONTACT EMS IMMEDIATELY!

Call the Poison Center at 800-222-1222

Swallowed Poison

Many substances are toxic, especially for young children. Medications, alcoholic beverages, cleaning supplies, chemicals, cosmetics, mouthwash, and some plants are just a few of the toxic substances children may encounter.

- Call EMS.
- Put on non-latex gloves and remove traces of the poisonous substance from the child's mouth with a napkin or tissue. Check the mouth carefully, including the roof of the mouth, and remove what you can see. **Do not** "sweep" the back of the throat with your finger, as this could push the substance farther into the child's throat.
- While waiting for EMS to arrive, call the Poison Center at 800-222-1222. Have the following information available:
  » Child's age and weight
  » What was swallowed (have the container or plant with you to describe)
  » Amount swallowed
  » Time that substance was swallowed
  » Child's condition
- Follow instructions from the Poison Center.

Observe the child for breathing difficulties (shortness of breath, wheezing, coughing). If the child stops breathing, begin rescue breathing while waiting for EMS personnel to arrive.
See "RESCUE BREATHING" for more information.

- If the child vomits and becomes unresponsive or unconscious, place the child on his side to prevent choking.
- When EMS personnel arrive:
  » Be prepared to provide detailed information regarding the poisoning situation.
  » Give them the product container or a piece of the plant swallowed.
  » If the child vomits, give EMS a sample of the vomit.

Inhaled Poison

Poisoning from inhaled fumes, such as carbon monoxide, can be life-threatening. Poisoning can also occur by inhaling fumes from substances such as rubber cement, model glue, or petroleum products.

- Remove the child (and everyone else) from the toxic area. This may require evacuation from the building.
- Call EMS.
- While waiting for EMS to arrive, call the Poison Center at 800-222-1222. Have the following information available:
  » Child's age and weight
  » What was inhaled
  » Time that substance was inhaled
  » Child's condition
- Follow instructions from the Poison Center.
- Contact the child's family.

Observe the child for breathing difficulties (shortness of breath, wheezing, coughing). If the child stops breathing, begin rescue breathing while waiting for EMS personnel to arrive. *See "RESCUE BREATHING" for more information.*

Skin Contact (irritating chemicals or substances)

Some substances, such as cleaning chemicals, can cause skin irritation.

- Immediately and thoroughly wash the area with soap and running water.
- Call the Poison Center at 800-222-1222.
- Follow instructions from the Poison Center. **Do not** follow any emergency instructions printed on product labels. Labels may be out-of-date or have incorrect treatment information.
- If the skin appears burned or the child is in pain, call EMS. *See "BURNS" for more information on treating chemical burns.*
- Contact the child's family.

Poison Ivy, Poison Oak, or Other Plants

Certain plants, such as poison ivy, poison oak, or sumac, can cause reactions. If contact with one of these plants is suspected:

- Immediately and thoroughly wash the area with soap and running water.
- Contact the child's family and inform them of the possible exposure.

PR℞ESCRIPTION FOR PREVENTION

- Store all medications in locked cabinets, out of children's reach.
- Store potentially toxic substances, such as cleaning supplies, out of reach and in areas that are inaccessible to children.
- Inspect play areas and carefully remove potentially harmful or toxic plants.

Allergic Reactions

Children can have allergic reactions to almost any substance, including medications, latex, insect stings, pollen, mold, food, or environmental "triggers" such as smoke, perfumes, or aerosols. Most reactions are mild. However, serious reactions can be life-threatening.

Anaphylaxis (severe allergic reaction)

Anaphylaxis is a **life-threatening problem** caused by a severe allergic reaction to a substance, such as exposure to a food (such as peanuts) or an insect bite or sting. Symptoms can occur quickly.

- Call EMS if the child has been exposed to a food, insect sting, medication, or other substance that has triggered a severe reaction in the past.
- Call EMS if you observe symptoms of serious reaction (anaphylaxis), such as:
  » Rash or hives on the body
  » Itching, including in the mouth
  » Swelling of the face, lips, tongue, or throat
  » Swelling of the body part where the sting or bite occurred (more than just minor swelling of the skin where stung/bitten)
  » Difficulty swallowing or speaking
  » Dizziness, unexplained confusion, fainting, or loss of consciousness
  » Breathing problems (shortness of breath, wheezing, coughing)
  » Abdominal pain, nausea, vomiting, or other sudden illness
- Be prepared to administer rescue breathing if necessary while waiting for EMS personnel to arrive. *See "RESCUE BREATHING" for more information.*
- A child who has had a previous severe reaction may have a doctor-prescribed auto-injector of epinephrine (such as EpiPen Jr or Twinject). Injectable epinephrine should be administered only if prescribed for that child by a physician.

Auto-Injector of Epinephrine (such as EpiPen Jr or Twinject)

- Epinephrine should not be used unless prescribed by the child's physician.
- If prescribed, the auto-injector **must** be kept near the child at all times.
- Store the auto-injector at room temperature in a safe, dry place. Check expiration date frequently. **Note**: Do not allow the auto-injector to freeze or overheat, or it will not be effective.
- Caregivers should be trained by medical personnel in correct use of the auto-injector.

To use an auto-injector:

- Hold the auto-injector in your hand and make a fist around it.
- Remove the safety cap.

- Place the black tip of the injector near the fleshy part of the child's outer thigh. (You can inject through the child's clothing.) **Do not** inject into the vein or the buttocks.
- With a rapid motion, push the auto-injector firmly against the thigh and hold it in place until the medication is injected, about 10 seconds. *See figure 10.*
- Remove the auto-injector; replace it into the safety tube or other container.
- Call EMS.
- Give the auto-injector to EMS personnel.

Mild Allergic Reactions

Mild allergic reactions may include redness of skin; itching, stuffy, or runny nose; sneezing; and itchy or watery eyes.

- If possible, remove the allergen or irritant.
    - » If the trigger is environmental (such as perfume or smoke), remove the child from the area.
    - » If the reaction is caused by skin contact with a substance, wash the child's skin with warm, soapy water.
- Observe the child for symptoms of serious allergic reaction. *See the Anaphylaxis section on the previous page for more information.*
- Refer to the child's medical record for information about previous allergic reactions.
    - » If the child has a prescribed health care plan, follow those instructions.
    - » Call EMS if the child has been exposed to a food, insect sting, medication, or other substance that has triggered a severe reaction in the past.
    - » A child who has had a previous severe reaction may have doctor-prescribed injectable epinephrine (such as EpiPen Jr or Twinject). *See the Anaphylaxis section on the previous page for more information on injectable epinephrine.*
    - » Contact the child's family and recommend medical attention.
    - » Families should notify the child's doctor of any reaction, especially a reaction to medication. The next exposure to the substance might result in a more severe reaction.
- Continue to observe the child for symptoms of serious allergic reaction, including breathing problems or **shock.** *See the section on Shock under "SUDDEN ILLNESS" for more information.*

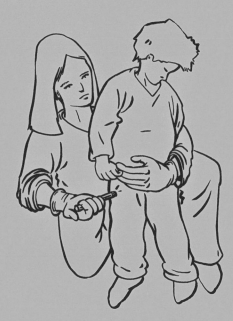

figure 10

<table>
<tr><td colspan="1" align="center">**PRₓESCRIPTION FOR PREVENTION**</td></tr>
</table>

- Document all allergies children have. Be sure all staff members are aware of potential allergy triggers.
- If a child is severely allergic to a substance such as peanuts, create a "peanut-free" environment. This means no products are allowed in the facility that contain peanuts or peanut byproducts. Most serious food-allergic reactions are from peanuts, tree nuts, fish, and shellfish.
- Avoid children's exposure to aerosols or fragranced air fresheners, cleaners, perfumes, and smoke.

Bites and Stings

Animal Bite

- Control bleeding with direct pressure. *See "BLEEDING" for more information.*
- Wash the wound area with soap and water.
- If the **skin is broken**, contact the child's family and recommend immediate medical attention.
- If the **skin is not broken**, apply a cloth-wrapped cold pack to the bruised area and comfort the child.
- Document all details of the incident, including the following information:
  - » Description of the animal that bit the child
  - » Location of the animal (including owner's name and address, if known)
  - » Date of the animal's last rabies vaccination, if known
  - » Any recent unusual behavior by the animal

CALL EMS IF:

- The child was bitten by a wild or stray animal; an animal whose rabies vaccination status is unknown; or an animal that is acting strangely.
- The child was bitten on the face, neck, or hand, or near a joint.
- The wound is deep.
- There are several bites.

Human Bite

Infants and toddlers put their mouths on people and toys, and many toddlers try biting. Most bites are not medically serious. However, there is a risk of infection if the skin is broken.

- Step in between the children to prevent further biting. Stay calm; do not raise your voice.
- Help the child who was bitten.

If the **skin is broken**:

- Control bleeding (if any).
- Wash the wound with soap and water.
- Apply a cloth-wrapped cold pack to the bite area.
- Comfort the child.
- Contact the child's family.
- Recommend the child's family check with their health care provider about additional care.

If the **skin is not broken**:

- Apply a cloth-wrapped cold pack to the bite area.
- Comfort the child.

Insect Bite or Sting

Most bites and stings cause mild reactions.

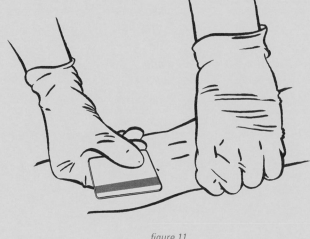

figure 11

- Inspect the affected area. Remove any body parts of the stinging or biting insect that may remain on or in the child's skin.
  - » Remove a stinger by scraping it with a plastic card (such as a credit card) or fingernail. *See figure 11.* Gently scrape it out from the same direction that it went into the skin. **Do not** use tweezers or squeeze the stinger.
  - » Remove caterpillar spines from a child's skin with sticky tape.
- Wash the area with soap and water.
- Apply a cloth-wrapped cold pack to reduce pain and swelling.
- If the bite involves the limbs (arms, legs), then keep the area elevated. (Example: If the hand is stung, raise the child's hand/arm so it is higher than the level of child's heart.)
- Observe the child for any symptoms of serious reaction. *See the section on Anaphylaxis under "ALLERGIC REACTIONS" for more information.* Any child can have a serious reaction to a sting or to multiple stings, even if the child has had no previous allergic reaction.

Spider Bite

Most spiders are venomous. Most spider bites cause mild reactions. However, bites from certain spiders can be serious and even life-threatening.

- Wash the bite area with soap and water.
- Apply a cloth-wrapped cold pack to reduce pain and swelling.
- Call the Poison Center at 800-222-1222 for further instruction.
- Contact the child's family and recommend medical attention if there is significant swelling or redness.

Call EMS if you suspect the bite is from a black widow or brown recluse spider. It will be helpful to EMS personnel if you can describe the spider or if you can catch or kill the spider (without squashing it beyond recognition).

Tick Bite

- Remove the tick as quickly as possible.
- Use tweezers to grasp the tick near its head, close to the child's skin. *See figure 12.*
  - » Gently pull in the direction from which the tick entered the skin.
  - » Continue gentle pressure for several seconds, until the tick lets go.
  - » **Do not** twist or jerk the tick. **Do not** rupture the tick's body.
- Wash the bite area with soap and water.
- After removing the tick:
  - » Keep the tick in a dry plastic bag or container for possible identification. (**Do not** put it in a container with rubbing alcohol or water.)
  - » Inform the child's family that you have removed a tick from the child.
  - » Wood tick bites are common but rarely cause additional health problems. However, bites from deer ticks can transmit Lyme disease. If a deer tick is suspected *(see figure 12-a)*, strongly recommend the child's family consult their health care provider's office for further instruction.

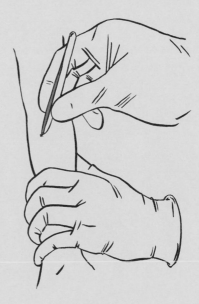

figure 12

Scorpion Sting

Scorpion stings may cause localized pain that increases rapidly. The pain may travel up the limb (arm or leg) that was stung. A child may have a severe reaction, including breathing problems, paralysis, or spasms.

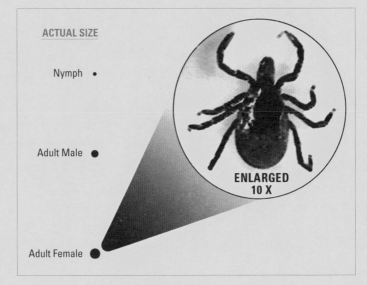

ACTUAL SIZE

Nymph •

Adult Male ●

Adult Female ●

ENLARGED
10 X

figure 12-a

- Call EMS.
- Wash the sting area with soap and water.
- Apply a cloth-wrapped cold pack.
- Notify the child's family of the sting.
- Observe the child for signs of serious reaction. *See the section on Anaphylaxis under "ALLERGIC REACTIONS" for more information.*

Snake Bite

- Call EMS.
- Wash the area with soap and water.
- Keep the child calm and the body part still. Keep the bitten area *lower* than the heart level.
- **Do not** apply an ice pack to a snake bite.
- Call the Poison Center at 800-222-1222 for advice. It will be helpful if you can describe the snake. However, **do not** try to catch the snake.
- Notify the child's family of the bite.
- Observe the child for signs of serious reaction. *See the section on Anaphylaxis under "ALLERGIC REACTIONS" for more information.*

PRₓESCRIPTION FOR PREVENTION

- Enclose outdoor play areas with fencing; keep gates securely latched.
- Keep outdoor play areas clean and free of trash, garbage, or debris.
- Check outdoor play area and play equipment each day for insect nests, spiderwebs, ant hills, and so on.

Burns

Thermal Burns (burns due to contact with a hot surface, hot liquid, fire, and so on)

- Run cool water over the burned skin.
- Continue to cool the skin with water until the pain stops or the child gets medical attention.
- Burns, even mild burns, can cause swelling. Remove any potentially constricting items in the burn area, such as rings or bracelets, if they can be *easily* removed. **Do not** attempt to remove items if removal is difficult or may cause further injury to the skin and tissue.
- **Do not** attempt to remove clothing or jewelry that may be stuck to the burned skin.
- **Do not** apply butter, ointment, cream, or lotion to the burned area.

CALL EMS IF:

- The burn involves the face, scalp, hands, feet, or genitals.
- The burn covers more than 1 percent of the body area (burn area is larger than the palm of the burn victim's hand).
- The burn area is raw, ash white, black, leathery, or charred.
- Clothing or jewelry is stuck to the burned skin.
- Child shows symptoms of **shock**. *See the section on Shock under "SUDDEN ILLNESS" for more information.*

Chemical Burns

- Brush off any dry chemicals from the skin.
- Rinse the affected skin with cool running water.
- Call EMS.
- Continue to rinse the area for at least 15 minutes while waiting for EMS to arrive.
- Call the Poison Center at 800-222-1222. Have the following information available:
  - » Child's age and weight
  - » Chemical substance or ingredients (have the container with you to describe)
  - » Area of body/skin affected
  - » Amount of chemical
  - » Time exposure occurred
  - » Child's condition, including description of skin
- Follow instructions from the Poison Center. Do not follow any emergency instructions printed on product labels. Labels may be out-of-date or have incorrect treatment information.
- Remove contaminated clothing.
  - » Avoid spreading the chemical to other areas of the child's body. **Do not** remove a contaminated shirt by pulling it over the child's head.
  - » If necessary, carefully cut clothing to remove it easily.

» **Do not** attempt to remove clothing that is stuck to the child's skin.
- Remove any potentially constricting items in the burn area, such as rings or bracelets, if they can be easily removed. **Do not** attempt to remove items if removal is difficult or may cause further injury to the skin and tissue.
- If the chemical burned the eye, call EMS and flush the eye gently with water for 15 minutes or until EMS arrives.

Electrical Burns

- Remove the child from the electrical source.
    - » Turn off the power source *before* touching the child.
    - » If power cannot be turned off, push or pull the child away from the source with an object that does not conduct electricity (such as a wooden or plastic object or a thickly folded *dry* cloth).
    - » **Do not** touch the child directly.
- Call EMS.
- Check the child for breathing. If necessary, begin rescue breathing. *See "RESCUE BREATHING" for more information.*
- Observe child for symptoms of shock. *See the section on Shock under "SUDDEN ILLNESS" for more information.*

PR_XESCRIPTION FOR PREVENTION

- Do not allow children access to hot appliances.
- Turn hot water thermostats to 120° F or lower.
- Cover all electrical outlets when not in use.
- Inspect and replace worn or frayed appliance cords.
- Teach children to "Stop, Drop, and Roll" to put out clothing that has caught on fire and practice the procedure.

Head, Neck, and Spine Injuries

Injury to the head, neck, or spine (back) requires **immediate** medical attention.

CALL EMS IF:

- The injury resulted from a fall, a blow to the head or back, a vehicle crash, or another significant force (which could impact the head, neck, or spine).
- You observe or the child complains of any of the following symptoms as a result of a head, neck, or spine injury:
  - » Unconsciousness, even if only for a few seconds
  - » Bleeding from any part of the head
  - » Bleeding or fluid from the nose, ear, or mouth
  - » Unusual sleepiness or listlessness
  - » "Goose egg" or swelling, especially of an infant's fontanel ("soft spot")
  - » Pale, sweaty appearance
  - » Seizure
  - » Severe headache
  - » Neck pain or stiffness; pain radiating through the shoulders
  - » Vomiting more than once
  - » Loss of bladder or bowel control
  - » Difficulty walking or moving arms or legs
  - » Dizziness, weakness, or paralysis
  - » Blurred vision
  - » Confusion or memory loss
  - » Slurred or difficult speech

Notify the child's family.

IF SEVERE INJURY IS SUSPECTED:

- **Do not** move the child while waiting for EMS to arrive.
- Calm the child and encourage the child to remain still.
- Observe the child for breathing problems (shortness of breath, wheezing, coughing).
- If the child stops breathing and rescue breathing is necessary, use the jaw-thrust method to open airway. Avoid tilting or moving the head and neck. *See "RESCUE BREATHING" for more information.*

Bone and Muscle Injuries

(When head, neck, or spine injury is not suspected.)

Bone and muscle injuries (sprain, strain, fracture, or dislocation) require medical attention.

- Stop the activity immediately.

CALL EMS IF:

- There is obvious swelling of the injured joint or area.
- There is an abnormal shape or position of the area (an arm or leg is at an unnatural angle or position, for example).
- The suspected bone/muscle injury involves an open wound.
- The child complains of significant pain when the injured part is touched or moved.
- The child shows symptoms of shock. *See the section on Shock under "SUDDEN ILLNESS" for more information.*
- **Do not** move the injured part while waiting for EMS to arrive.
  - » **Do not** move the child (unless the child is in immediate danger of further injury).
  - » **Do not** encourage the child to move the injured body part or "walk it off."
  - » **Do not** attempt to "straighten" or "relocate" the injured limb or joint.
  - » **Do not** attempt to apply a splint or compression bandage. This level of treatment should be administered by a trained health care professional.
- Contact the child's family.

If the injury appears to be minor and EMS is **not** called:

- Have the child sit or lie in a comfortable position.
- Help the child keep the injured part still if movement causes pain.
- Apply a cloth-wrapped cold pack for 20 minutes every hour.
- Elevate the injured part (if arm or leg) above the level of the heart by supporting on pillows or blankets.
- Contact the child's family and explain the nature of the injury. Recommend that the family seek medical attention for the child.

11

PRₓESCRIPTION FOR PREVENTION

- Install approved resilient surfacing under and around all play equipment. *See "RESOURCES" for more information on the U.S. Consumer Product Safety Commission's Handbook for Public Playground Safety.*
- Require that each child wear a helmet when playing on wheeled toys.
- Install secure child-level handrails for all stairways. Install a non-slip surface on steps and ramps.
- Keep pathways clear. Provide adequate lighting.

Heat-Related Conditions

Heat Exhaustion

Heat exhaustion can occur when a person gets too hot, loses fluid by sweating, and doesn't consume enough fluids (dehydration).

- Observe the child for symptoms of heat exhaustion, including:
  - » Weakness or dizziness
  - » Complaints of nausea
  - » Complaints of painful muscle spasms. *See section on Heat Cramps on the next page for more information.*
- Move the child to a cool place.
- If a cool place is not available, cool the child's body with wet, cool cloths or pour cool water over his skin.
- Encourage the child to sip water.
- Observe the child for symptoms of **heat stroke** or **dehydration**. *See the Heat Stroke section below and the Dehydration section on the next page for more information.*

CALL EMS IF:

- The child's body temperature rises. *See "FEVER" for more information on taking a child's temperature.*
- You observe any symptoms of heat stroke. *See the Heat Stroke section below for more information.*
- The child shows symptoms of shock. *See the section on Shock under "SUDDEN ILLNESS" for more information.*
- The child does not feel better in a few minutes.

Heat Stroke

Heat stroke is life-threatening! The child's body temperature increases and can quickly reach 108° F or higher. The child must be cooled *quickly* to avoid permanent brain damage.

Call EMS. This is a life-threatening emergency!

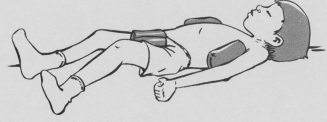

figure 13

- Move the child to a cool place.
- Immediately remove unnecessary clothing from the child.
- Pour cool water over the child's head and body, or place the child in a tub of cool or cold water. Avoid getting water in the child's nose or mouth.
- Place cloth-wrapped cold packs in the child's armpits and groin. *See figure 13.*

- If child is awake, give him sips of cool water.
- If child vomits and is unconscious, turn the child's body to the side to prevent choking.

OBSERVE THE CHILD FOR SYMPTOMS OF HEAT STROKE, INCLUDING:

- Hot, red, and unusually dry skin (no sweating)
- Elevated body temperature (fever) *See "FEVER" for more information on taking a child's temperature.*
- Rapid heartbeat
- Breathing problems (shortness of breath, wheezing, coughing)
- Headache
- Weakness, dizziness, fainting
- Confusion or decreasing level of responsiveness

Heat Cramps

Heat cramps are brief, severe cramps in the leg, arm, or abdomen that can occur after playing in hot weather or a hot environment. They are painful but not serious.

- Move the child to a cool place.
- Encourage the child to drink water.
- Gently massage the painful area.
- Observe the child for symptoms of heat exhaustion, heat stroke, or dehydration.

Dehydration

Dehydration occurs when a child doesn't drink enough water or fluid to replace the fluid lost from perspiration, urination, diarrhea, or vomiting.

- Observe the child for symptoms of dehydration, including:
  » Dry skin and mouth
  » Sunken eyes
  » Failure to urinate within 6 daytime hours of last urination; urine is dark in color
  » Crying with few tears
- Encourage the child to drink liquids, including:
  » Water
  » Oral rehydration solutions such as Pedialyte
- **Do not** give milk, salty broths, fruit juices, or carbonated beverages.
- Call EMS. Dehydration can be very dangerous, especially for infants and young children.

Sunburn

- Remove the child from sun exposure. Move the child to a cool place.
- Skin may be red and abnormally warm. Child may complain of pain.
- Apply cool compresses to relieve pain.
- Do not apply ointments or lotions (unless you have written authorization and lotion is prescribed specifically for that child).

- Observe the child for symptoms of heat-related illness.
  - » Call EMS if the child's body temperature is elevated (fever). This can indicate **heat stroke**, a life-threatening problem.
  - » Encourage the child to sip water. Observe the child for signs of dehydration.
- Contact the child's family and recommend medical attention if:
  - » An infant under one year of age is sunburned.
  - » The sunburned skin includes fluid-filled blisters.
  - » The child is in severe pain.
  - » There is swelling related to the sunburn, especially around the eyes.

PR$_X$ESCRIPTION FOR PREVENTION

- Be aware of heat and UV index for outdoor play. Plan indoor, air-conditioned activities during the sunniest part of summer days.
- Encourage children to play in the shade.
- Help children dress appropriately for warm weather. Removable layers are best.
- Provide plenty of water and encourage children to drink frequently throughout the day.
- Do not leave children unattended in vehicles.
- Recommend families provide sunscreen to prevent sunburn.

Cold-Related Conditions

Frostnip

Frostnip is a nonfreezing injury of the skin tissues, usually of the fingers, toes, ears, cheeks, and chin. It is the most common cold injury. Symptoms of frostnip include:

- Reddened, gray, or pale skin
- Stiff-feeling skin with soft and resilient underlying tissue. If a person presses against the tissue, the skin indentation springs back.
- Injured tissues that turn pink or even red as the body part is warmed
- Indications from the child of numbness or tingling as skin is warmed

Frostnip can occur if ice or a cold pack is placed directly on a child's skin. Always wrap ice packs or cold packs in a soft cloth, or place a cloth or towel between the child's skin and the cold pack.

- Take the child to a warm place. If a warm place is not immediately available, place cold body parts close to warm body areas (tuck cold hands into armpits, for example).
- Allow cold-injured parts to *slowly* return to normal body temperature.
- **Do not** rub affected areas.
- Keep the child warm. Prevent refreezing of area, which could cause severe tissue damage.
- Contact the child's family and recommend they contact their physician for further instruction.

Frostbite

Frostbite is tissue damage caused by freezing of the body tissue. The ears, face, hands, and feet are most likely to be affected.

- Call EMS.
- Observe child for symptoms of frostbite, including:
  - » Injured skin appears pale or bluish.
  - » Skin and tissue may feel cold, solid, and woodlike. If a person presses against the tissue, the skin indentation **does not** spring back.
  - » Child indicates her skin feels numb.
  - » Injured skin may have small blisters containing either clear or bloody fluid.
  - » As the body part is warmed, injured tissues may turn pink or red. If damage is severe, tissue may remain pale.
  - » Injured tissue may hurt, tingle, or feel like it is burning as it warms.
- Take the child to a warm place. If a warm place is not immediately available, place cold body parts close to warm body areas (tuck cold hands into armpits, for example).
- Remove wet clothes, shoes, and socks. Dress the child in clean, dry clothes or wrap her in a warm blanket.
- Allow cold-injured parts to *slowly* return to normal body temperature.

- **Do not** rub affected areas. **Do not** rub area with snow.
- If fingers or toes are cold-damaged, put dry gauze between the fingers/toes.
- If blisters are present, cover with gauze. Do not break blisters.
- Contact the child's family.

Hypothermia

Hypothermia occurs when the core body temperature drops below 95° F. Hypothermia is often caused by falling into cold water or being outside too long without protective clothing.

- Call EMS.
- Observe the child for symptoms of hypothermia, including:
  » A lower-than-normal body temperature
  » Confusion or unresponsiveness
  » Unconsciousness
- Warm the child quickly. Take the child to a warm place. If a warm place is not immediately available, hold the child close to someone else's warm body.
- Remove wet clothes, shoes, and socks. Dress the child in warm, dry clothes or wrap in a warm blanket.
- Keep the child wrapped in a blanket while waiting for EMS to arrive.
- Contact the child's family.

PR℞ESCRIPTION FOR PREVENTION

- Help children dress appropriately for cold weather. Removable layers are best.
- Limit children's time outside in very cold weather. If there is a combination of severe cold and wind chill, plan indoor activities.

Convulsions and Seizures

CALL EMS IF:

- The child has breathing difficulties (shortness of breath, wheezing, coughing).
- The child has no known seizure history.
- You do not have a seizure care plan for the child.
- The child remains unconscious or unresponsive after a seizure.
- The child falls or hits his head during a seizure.

FOR OTHER CONVULSIONS AND SEIZURES:

- Gently place the child on the floor or ground.
- If the child is drooling or vomits, position the child on his side.
- Loosen tight-fitting clothing around head or neck.
- Remove nearby objects (such as furniture and toys).
- Protect the child's head from impact by sliding the palm of your hand, a towel, or a blanket under the child's head. *See figure 14.*
- **Do not** put your fingers or any object in the mouth of a child during a seizure.
- Observe the child for breathing. Perform rescue breathing if necessary. *See "RESCUE BREATHING" for more information.*
- Document the time the seizure begins and ends. Provide a detailed description of the episode to the family and medical personnel. Notice which extremities are involved (one side, both sides, arm and/or leg, for example). Note if the child had a fever or acted ill before the seizure.

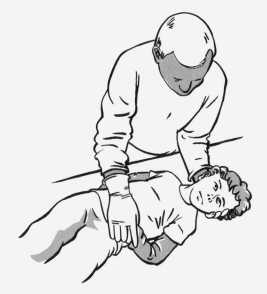

figure 14

14

Sudden Illness

Shock

Shock is a life-threatening condition that causes very low, inadequate blood pressure. Shock occurs because the body is not getting enough blood flow. It can occur as a reaction to illness or injury, such as bleeding, internal injury, dehydration, or allergic reaction.

Call EMS. **Shock requires immediate medical treatment** and can get worse very rapidly.

OBSERVE THE CHILD FOR SYMPTOMS OF SHOCK, INCLUDING:

- Pale, cool, or clammy skin
- Weak, rapid pulse
- Shallow breathing
- Unresponsiveness or unconsciousness
- If the child is conscious, he or she may feel faint, very weak, or confused.

TREATMENT AND PREVENTION OF SHOCK INCLUDE:

- Calming the child.
- Keeping the child warm (not hot) and as comfortable as possible. Loosen tight clothing.
- Having the child lie down on her back with feet higher than the head. If raising the legs will cause pain or further injury, keep the child flat.
- Observing the child for breathing problems.

Fainting

Fainting is a sudden and temporary loss of responsiveness caused by a brief lack of adequate blood and oxygen to the brain.

- Evaluate the situation and determine a possible cause for the fainting, such as:
  - » The child has not eaten sufficiently.
  - » The child reacted to a situation (stress, fear of needles, or sight of blood, for example).
  - » The child reacted to pain.
  - » The child overexerted herself physically or became too hot.
  - » The child has been standing too long.
  - » The child was holding her breath during a crying episode.
- Call EMS if the fainting is associated with:
  - » An injury, particularly a head injury
  - » Illness or fever
  - » Pain
  - » Allergic reaction

15

» Heat stroke
» Bleeding

- Lay the child on her back to prevent falling.
- Elevate the legs 8 to 12 inches.
- Loosen tight-fitting clothing.
- Observe the child for breathing difficulties (shortness of breath, wheezing, coughing). Perform rescue breathing if necessary. *See "RESCUE BREATHING" for more information.*

CALL EMS IF:

- The child remains unresponsive for more than a minute or so after elevating her legs.
- The child fell while fainting and possibly received a blow to the head.
- The child becomes blue or pale.

Diabetic Reaction/Hypoglycemia

IF A CHILD IS DIAGNOSED WITH DIABETES OR ANOTHER CHRONIC CONDITION:

- ECE staff members should work with the child's health care professionals to develop an emergency care plan.
- Any prescribed medications or supplies (such as glucose monitors or insulin) must be kept near the child at all times. Medications must be properly stored and out of children's reach.
- Caregivers directly involved in the care of the child must have specific training related to the child's condition, including administration of medication and emergency care.
- Other staff members involved in the care of the child should be aware of the condition and that there is an emergency care plan.
- Maintain written authorization forms of when and how to check the child's blood sugar levels.

Hypoglycemia (low blood sugar level) is one of the most frequent complications of diabetes. It can happen very suddenly and is not always preventable. Most hypoglycemic episodes are mild.

Symptoms may include the following:

- Headache
- Shakiness or tremors
- Dizziness
- Increased heart rate or palpitations
- Pale skin
- Clammy skin or sweating
- Lethargy
- Changing level of responsiveness, including mood changes

Treatment for hypoglycemia:

- Have the child eat or drink fast-acting carbohydrates, such as fruit juice, fruit beverage, crackers, or other food as indicated in the child's emergency care plan.
- Follow the child's emergency care plan, including contacting the child's family or EMS if indicated.

Abdominal Pain

Mild abdominal pain may be due to a number of causes, including overeating and intestinal gas. Severe abdominal pain, or pain accompanied by other symptoms, may indicate serious illness or injury.

- Contact the child's family and recommend medical attention if you observe or the child complains of these symptoms:
  - » Severe abdominal pain
  - » Localized pain (such as pain on one side)
  - » Pain accompanied by vomiting or fever
  - » Bloody stools (bowel movement)
  - » Pain after a fall or blow to the abdomen
- **Do not** give the child anything to eat or drink.
- Testicular (scrotal) pain is often described by children as abdominal pain.
  - » Scrotal pain is a medical emergency.
  - » Contact the child's family and recommend medical attention.

Other Symptoms That May Indicate Illness or Injury

If you observe or the child complains of these or other symptoms, contact the child's family and recommend medical attention.

- Unexplained pain
- Stiffness of the neck
- Vomiting and/or diarrhea, especially in combination with fever or other symptoms
- Lethargy, listlessness
- Sudden onset of rash
- Unexplainable confusion
- Looking or acting severely ill
- Unexpected behavior or mood swings

Young children do not always respond to pain or discomfort as expected. A child may have a serious injury, such as a broken bone, and yet not complain or show pain or discomfort.

Adults often have intuition about the children in their care. If you think a child has an illness or injury, even if there are no obvious symptoms, contact the child's family. As appropriate, recommend or arrange for a child's health care. **Do not** ignore your intuition!

Fever

Fever is a body temperature that is higher than normal. The average normal body temperature is 98.6° F.

- Observe the child for symptoms of fever, including:
  » A flushed face
  » Hot skin that may be dry or sweaty
  » Body (forehead, abdomen, back) that feels hot
- Evaluate the situation and determine a possible cause for the fever, such as:
  » The child (especially an infant) being dressed or covered too warmly. Remove unnecessary blankets and/or clothing.
  » An environment that is too warm (children playing outside in warm weather, for example). Move the child to a cooler environment. Observe the child for symptoms of heat exhaustion or heat stroke. *See "HEAT-RELATED CONDITIONS" for more information.*
  » A recent vaccination. A fever may occur within the first 24 to 48 hours.
  » An illness or infection. Observe the child for additional symptoms of illness or injury.
- Take the child's temperature. *See the section on Taking a Child's Temperature on the following pages for more information.*
  » Electronic ear thermometers are recommended for infants over 3 months of age and children.
  » Recorded body temperature may vary depending upon how the temperature is taken. Axillary temperature (under the arm) generally registers approximately 1 degree lower than tympanic (ear) temperature.
- If thermometer reading indicates normal body temperature (98.6° F):
  » Continue to observe the child for symptoms of fever or other illness or injury.
  » Continue to evaluate the environment and eliminate cause of overheating (child overdressed, room too hot, child playing outdoors on hot day).
  » Prevent dehydration. Offer infants breast milk or formula. Offer water to older children. *See "HEAT-RELATED CONDITIONS" for more information on dehydration.*
  » If symptoms persist, contact the child's family.

Response to Elevated Body Temperature (fever)

(NOTE: Normal body temperature is 98.6° F if measured with an ear thermometer. Axillary [under the arm] temperature is approximately 97.6° F—or 1 degree less than normal body temperature.) *See the section on Taking a Child's Temperature on the following pages for more information.*

- Young infant (age 3 months or younger):
  » An axillary temperature over 99.4° F indicates a need for medical attention.
  » Contact the child's family and recommend medical attention.
- Infant (age 4 to 12 months):
  » Oral or ear temperature of 102° F or higher indicates a need for medical attention.

» Contact the child's family and recommend medical attention.
- Toddler or older child:
  » Oral or ear temperature of 102° F or higher indicates a need for medical attention.
  » Contact the child's family and recommend medical attention.
- **Do not** give medication to lower temperature.

Fever is not a disease; it is a symptom. Fever accompanied by other symptoms may indicate a serious or life-threatening condition.

CALL EMS IF FEVER IS ACCOMPANIED BY OTHER SYMPTOMS, INCLUDING:

- Seizure or convulsions
- Stiff neck
- Irregular breathing
- Symptoms of heat stroke *See "HEAT-RELATED CONDITIONS" for more information.*

Contact the child's family and recommend medical attention if fever is accompanied by other symptoms, including:

- Fussiness, changing level of responsiveness, or unusual sleepiness
- Confusion
- Rash
- Ear pain (child is tugging on his ear)
- Persistent sore throat
- Vomiting and/or diarrhea
- Painful, burning, or frequent urination

Types of Thermometers

Caregivers should be trained in the proper use of a thermometer.

- Electronic ear thermometers (also called tympanic or aural thermometers):
  » These are quick, accurate, and easy to use.
  » Always use a disposable thermometer cover.
  » Follow manufacturer's instructions for your specific thermometer. Store the instruction sheet with the thermometer.
  » Ear thermometers are not recommended for young infants (age 3 months or less) because the infant's ear canal is so small. Use an axillary (under arm) temperature taking method for very young infants.
- Temporal artery thermometers:
  » These electronic thermometers, which are rubbed gently across the temple and forehead, are quick, accurate, easy to use, and non-invasive.
  » Can be easily cleaned with alcohol between uses.
  » Follow manufacturer's instructions for your specific thermometer. Store the instruction sheet with the thermometer.
- Plastic digital thermometers:
  » These inexpensive thermometers are quick, accurate, and easy to use.
  » Always use a disposable thermometer cover.

» Response time varies, so it's best to select one that beeps when the child's temperature is recorded.
» Follow manufacturer's instructions for your specific thermometer. Store the instruction sheet with the thermometer.
» These can be used to measure temperature either axillary (under the arm) or oral (in the mouth).
- Plastic strip or "forehead thermometers" are small plastic strips that you press against the child's forehead. These may not be accurate and are not recommended.
- Pacifier thermometers may not be accurate and are not recommended.
- **Never** use a glass thermometer.

Taking a Child's Temperature

Caregivers should use non-invasive methods to measure a child's body temperature. Only trained caregivers should be allowed to take a child's temperature.

DIGITAL THERMOMETER

- Choose a digital thermometer. Make sure the digital thermometer is in the "ON" mode.
- Dry the child's armpit with a soft cloth.
- Place the thermometer in the child's armpit. Gently hold the arm down close to the child's body. *See figure 15.*
- Hold the child in this position until the digital thermometer beeps.
- Read the thermometer. Normal axillary temperature is 97.6° F (1 degree *less* than the normal body temperature of 98.6° F).

EAR THERMOMETER

- An ear thermometer is recommended for infants age 4 months and older, and for children.
- Follow manufacturer's instructions for use.

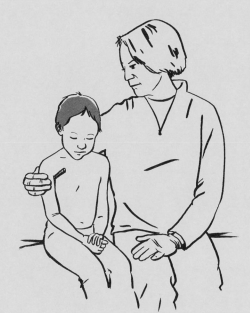

figure 15

OTHER CONSIDERATIONS

- **Do not** take a child's temperature rectally (in the bottom).
- Oral (mouth) temperature recordings are **not** recommended.
  The accuracy can be affected by the placement in the child's mouth, opening or breathing through the mouth, or if the child has eaten or drunk something hot or cold. Oral temperature should not be used for infants.
- **Never** use a glass thermometer.
- Use a disposable thermometer cover.

Taking an Infant's Temperature

For infants 3 months and under: Contact the child's family for permission to contact the child's health care provider for appropriate action. Make sure a Release of Information form has been signed and is on file.

For infants 4 months and over, and for toddlers: An electronic ear thermometer or temporal artery thermometer is recommended. Follow the manufacturer's instructions.

Dental Injuries

Injury to the Lip, Tongue, or Gums

- Put on non-latex gloves.
- Position the child to prevent blood from going down the airway. Help the child sit up with head tilted slightly forward, or lie on one side.
- Help the child rinse her mouth with water so you can identify the injured area.
- Apply direct pressure to the bleeding area with gauze or a clean cloth.
- Apply cold compresses to reduce swelling.
- Contact the child's family and recommend dental or medical care.

CALL EMS IF:

- Bleeding does not stop after 5 minutes of continuous direct pressure.
- The wound is deep or large.
- The wound cuts across the tongue.
- The wound involves the back or roof of the mouth or the throat.
- The wound involves the lip and face.
- The wound is from an animal bite.

Broken Tooth

- Put on non-latex gloves.
- Help the child rinse her mouth with water so you can identify the injured area.
- Give the child a cold compress to hold on the injured tooth, or hold a cold compress on her face in the area of the broken tooth.
- Collect all the pieces of the tooth. Put pieces in a cold, wet cloth or in a container (such as a plastic zipper bag) of water or milk.
- Call the child's family to arrange for immediate dental care.

Knocked-Out Tooth

- Put on non-latex gloves.
- Position the child to prevent blood from going down the airway. Help the child sit up with head tilted slightly forward, or lie on one side.
- Help the child rinse her mouth with water so you can identify the injured area.
- If bleeding, apply direct pressure to the area with gauze or a clean cloth.
- Give the child a cold compress to hold on the injured area, or hold a cold compress on her face in the area of the knocked-out tooth.
- Attempt to find the tooth. If you find the tooth:
  - » Hold the tooth by the crown (the top), not the root.
  - » Remove visible dirt by gently rinsing with water. Do not scrub the tooth.

- Keep the tooth moist.
  - » If there is concern that the child might swallow the tooth if you try to replace it, put the tooth in a cold, wet cloth or a container of water or milk.
  - » For an older child, and if the child can cooperate, replace the tooth gently in the socket, then have the child bite down on a gauze pad or cloth to keep it in place.
- Contact the child's family and arrange for *immediate* dental care. Professional dental care within 1 to 2 hours may save the tooth.
- Professional dental care is important, even if the knocked-out tooth cannot be found.

Toothache

A toothache may be a dental emergency (an abscessed or injured tooth, for example), or it may refer to more common discomfort associated with teething, mouth sores, earache or ear infection, or sinus infection. Toothaches may also be caused by food caught between the teeth.

- Put on non-latex gloves.
- Help the child rinse her mouth with water.
- If the child's toothbrush (or a new, clean toothbrush) is available, have the child brush her teeth thoroughly.
- If the child can cooperate, floss her teeth gently to remove any food that might be lodged between teeth.
  - » Break off about 18 inches of floss and wind most of it around one of your middle fingers. Wind the remaining floss around the same finger of the opposite hand. Hold the floss tightly between your thumbs and forefingers.
  - » Guide the floss between the teeth using a gentle rubbing motion.
  - » When the floss reaches the gum line, curve it into a C-shape against one tooth. Gently slide it into the space between the gum and the tooth.
  - » Hold the floss tightly against the tooth. Gently rub the side of the tooth, moving the floss away from the gum with back and forth motions.
- Again, help the child rinse her mouth with water. Removal of lodged food may alleviate the pain.

IF THE CHILD STILL COMPLAINS OF PAIN:

- Give the child a cold compress to hold on her face in the area of the toothache.
- Contact the child's family and recommend dental or medical care.
- Recommend immediate dental or medical care if:
  - » The pain is very severe.
  - » The child has a fever (over 100° F).
  - » The child's face is swollen.
  - » The child is acting very sick.

PRESCRIPTION FOR PREVENTION

- Keep pathways and children's play areas clear of debris to prevent falls.
- Keep supplies on hand for emergency tooth preservations. Two such products available are Save-A-Tooth and the EMT ToothSaver.

Eye, Ear, and Nose Emergencies

Eye Trauma

Eye trauma refers to any injury to the eye. Eye injury is the most common and preventable cause of blindness. Immediate medical attention is needed for any eye injury.

- Call EMS for any injury to the eye or the eye area.
- Call EMS if you observe or the child complains of any of the following symptoms related to the eye or vision:
  » Blood in the eye
  » Inability to open the eye after trauma
  » Pain when moving the eye
  » Redness and swelling of the eyelid
  » Extreme sensitivity to light
  » Double vision
  » Decrease in vision
  » Numbness in the eye

Chemical Injury to Eye

- Put on non-latex gloves.
- Immediately rinse the injured eye with water.
  » Have the child lie on one side (same side as injured eye). Place a towel under the child's head (to absorb water).
  » Hold the injured eye open. You may need assistance for this.
  » Using a cup or small pitcher, pour cool water over the injured eye. Flush with water so that water flows from inside corner (by nose) toward the outside corner of eye (toward the ear). *See figure 16.*
- Call EMS.
- Call the Poison Center at 800-222-1222.
- Continue rinsing the eye for at least 15 minutes or until EMS arrives.

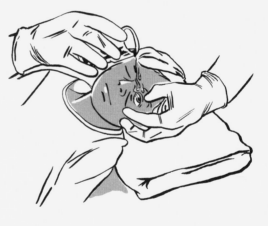

figure 16

Scratch, Cut, or Penetrating Injury to Eye or Eye Area

- Call EMS.
- Put on non-latex gloves.
- Keep the child as quiet as possible. It is best for the child to lie still, flat on his back, but do not force the child to lie down.

- If the child will cooperate, attempt to cover the eye with an eye shield or paper cup. This will help protect the eye.
- **Do not** apply any pressure to the eye.

Foreign Object in Eye (dust, sand)

- Put on non-latex gloves.
- Check for dust, sand, or another object in the eye if you observe or the child complains of any of the following symptoms:
  - » Rubbing the eye
  - » Watery or reddened eye
  - » Itching, or scratchy-feeling
  - » Pain
  - » Sensitivity to light
  - » Blurry vision
- Keep the child from pressing on or rubbing the eye.
- Gently examine the eye. *See figure 17.*
  - » Pull the lower lid down and ask the child to look up.
  - » Then hold the upper lid while the child looks down.
- If the object is obviously floating (moving) in the tear film on the surface of the eye, try flushing it out.
  - » Have the child lie on one side (same side as injured eye). Place a towel under the child's head (to absorb water).
  - » Hold the injured eye open. You may need assistance for this.
  - » Using a cup or small pitcher, pour cool water over the injured eye. Flush with water so that water flows from inside corner (by nose) toward the outside corner of eye (toward the ear).
- **Do not** try to remove an object except by flushing with water.
- **Do not** attempt to touch the object.
- Contact the child's family and recommend immediate medical attention (preferably an ophthalmologist or primary care physician) if:
  - » The object is not easily flushed out.
  - » The object appears to be embedded in the eye.
  - » The child continues to complain of pain, irritation, or blurred vision.
  - » The eye continues to be red, or swelling is present.

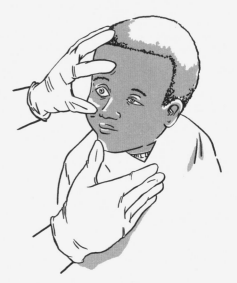

figure 17

Blunt Force Trauma to Eye or Eye Area (black eye)

- Gently apply cold compresses intermittently: 5 to 10 minutes on, 10 to 15 minutes off.
- Contact the child's family and recommend medical evaluation. Blunt force trauma (such as getting hit by a ball or a fist) can cause internal damage.

CALL EMS IF ANY OF THE FOLLOWING SYMPTOMS ARE OBSERVED:

- Drainage from the eye
- Any visible abnormality of the eyeball
- Visible bleeding on the white part of the eye

Contact the child's family and recommend *immediate* medical attention (preferably an ophthalmologist) if any of the following symptoms are observed:

- Increased redness
- Persistent eye pain
- Any changes in vision

Other Symptoms Related to Eyes and Vision

Contact the child's family and recommend medical attention if you observe or the child complains of any of the following symptoms:

- Redness, or "blood-shot" eyes
- Excessive rubbing of the eyes, itching, or irritation
- Discharge or "crusty" particles, especially after the child has been asleep
- Squinting or holding objects close to the face when playing

PR$_\text{X}$ESCRIPTION FOR PREVENTION

- Teach children to avoid throwing sand and dirt into the air.
- Keep all spray and aerosol substances out of children's reach.

Earache

Pain in or around the ear area may be caused by a variety of conditions, including ear infection (otitis media), teething, sinus infection, or other illness or injury.

- Symptoms of ear pain may include crying, fever, and fussiness—especially if child is also pulling or rubbing his ear.
- Contact the child's family and arrange for medical attention.

Foreign Object in Ear

A foreign object (such as a rock, insect, or bean) in the ear canal can cause pain and hearing loss.

- Using a flashlight or other bright light, look inside the child's ear canal.
- If the object is clearly visible, is flexible, and can be grasped easily with tweezers, gently remove it.
- If the object cannot be grasped with tweezers, tilt the child's head to the affected side and keep child still. Contact the child's family and arrange for medical attention.
- **Do not** probe the ear with a cotton swab, matchstick, or other tool. This could push the object farther into the ear.

Contact the child's family and recommend medical attention if:

- The object cannot be easily removed.
- The child continues to complain of pain after object is removed.

- There is bleeding in the ear.
- The ear continues to be red or swelling is present.
- The child appears to have hearing loss.

Foreign Object in Nose

Children sometimes insert objects, such as a rock or bean, in their noses.

- Contact the child's family and recommend medical attention.

Resources

American Academy of Pediatrics, *Healthy Child Care America,* www.healthychildcare.org.

American Academy of Pediatrics. *Pediatric First Aid for Caregivers and Teachers*. Sudbury, Mass.: Jones and Bartlett Publishers, 2007.

American Academy of Pediatrics, American Public Health Association, and National Resource Center for Health and Safety in Child Care and Early Education. *Caring for Our Children: National Health and Safety Performance Standards: Guidelines for Out-of-Home Child Care Programs,* 2nd edition. Elk Grove Village, Ill.: American Academy of Pediatrics and Washington, D.C.: American Public Health Association, 2002. Also available at http://nrc.uchsc.edu.

American Heart Association, www.americanheart.org.

American School Health Association's Council on Early Childhood Health Education and Services, *Healthy Childcare*, www.healthychild.net.

Aronson, Susan S. and Timothy R. Shope, eds. *Managing Infectious Diseases in Child Care and Schools: A Quick Reference Guide.* Elk Grove Village, Ill.: American Academy of Pediatrics, 2004.

Healthy Childcare Consultants, Inc., *Health and Safety Training Programs for Childcare Staff and Parents,* www.childhealthonline.org/strain.html.

Healthy Childcare Consultants, Inc., HIP on Health Parent Information Series, www.childhealthonline.org/parents.html.

National Child Care Health Consultant Registry, http://hcccnsc.edc.org/registry.

National Program for Playground Safety, www.uni.edu/playground.

National Resource Center for Health and Safety in Child Care and Early Education, *Healthy Kids, Healthy Care,* www.healthykids.us.

National Resource Center for Health and Safety in Child Care and Early Education, *Individual States' Child Care Licensure Regulations,* http://nrc.uchsc.edu/STATES/states.htm.

Smith, Connie Jo, Charlotte M. Hendricks, and Becky S. Bennett. *Growing, Growing Strong: A Whole Health Curriculum for Young Children.* St. Paul, Minn.: Redleaf Press, 2006.

U.S. Consumer Product Safety Commission. *Handbook for Public Playground Safety*. Washington, D.C.: 1997. Available for download at www.cpsc.gov/CPSCPUB/PUBS/325.pdf.

Credits

Author

Dr. Charlotte M. Hendricks

Dr. Hendricks is a Certified Health Education Specialist with over 25 years' experience in early childhood health education and research. She is the president of Healthy Childcare Consultants, Inc. (www.childhealthonline.org), editor for *Healthy CHILDCare Magazine*, and project director for the Sun Safety Alliance's SunSafe Childcare Project. A nationally recognized leader in health and safety education for child care and preschool, Dr. Hendricks is a recipient of the American School Health Association's Distinguished Service Award.

Medical Reviewers

Donald Palmer, MD
Magnolia Springs, AL

Hilary Pert Stecklein, MD
St. Paul, MN

Elaine Abrams, RN, CHES, MPH
Community Health Coordinator
Nursing & Home Care
Wilton, CT

Dianne Steudel Burdette, RN, BSN, CPN
Child Care Health Consultant Coordinator
The Children's Home Society of New Jersey

Sharis LeMay, RN, BNCSN
Assistant Director of Children's Health
Alabama Dept. of Public Health

Kathy Hunt, RDH
Healthy Smiles Community
Dental Hygiene Program
Wamego, KS

Marie Mitchell
Health Information Specialist
Pembroke, KY
Healthy Childcare Alabama
Alabama Dept. of Public Health

Debbie Parker, RN, BSN
Childcare Nurse Consultant
Healthy Childcare Alabama
Alabama Dept. of Public Health

Brenda Davis, RN
Childcare Nurse Consultant
Healthy Childcare Alabama
Alabama Dept. of Public Health

Daphne Pate, RN
Childcare Nurse Consultant
Healthy Childcare Alabama
Alabama Dept. of Public Health

Cyndy Henderson, RN, MSN
Childcare Nurse Consultant
Healthy Childcare Alabama
Alabama Dept. of Public Health

Published by Redleaf Press
10 Yorkton Court
St. Paul, MN 55117
www.redleafpress.org

First edition 2008
Cover design by Mayfly Design
Interior typeset and designed by Mayfly Design
Interior illustrations by Brian Trotter
Printed in the United States of America
15 14 13 12 11 10 09 08   1 2 3 4 5 6 7 8

Library of Congress Cataloging-in-Publication Data
Medical emergencies in early childhood settings. -- 1st ed.
    p. cm.
 ISBN 978-1-933653-62-4 (alk. paper)
 1. Pediatric emergencies--Handbooks, manuals, etc. 2. First aid in illness and injury--Hand-
books, manuals, etc. 3. Day care centers--Handbooks, manuals, etc. 4. Nursery schools--Hand-
books, manuals, etc.
 RJ370.M43 2008
 618.92'0025--dc22
                            2007046336

Printed on acid-free paper